Giving the Gift of
Receiving

Drake Kirkham

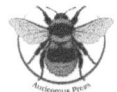

Library of Congress Control Number: 2024926231

ISBN 978-1-965067-05-5

Cover and interior design by Aubrey Bjork

Published Auricomus Press in Rexburg, Idaho
© 2024

With a diagnosis of Multiple Sclerosis (MS), I expected hardship; I have not been disappointed.

I've also received invaluable life lessons along with the challenges. One of the big ones is that giving yourself the grace to be more open allows more grace to flow into your life.

May these lessons both abound and astound you as they have me.

The tile was cold. Too cold. Or was it the shock beginning to settle in? Thoughts raced through my mind as I lay prostrate on our handicap-accessible bathroom floor—all six foot four of me. One minute I was struggling to slide across the board unaided, insisting grit would be enough to captain a sinking ship; the next, I had slid naked to the deck—through my wife's flailing arms—and lay flat, unable to move. Stuck, like a fish out of water, as a result of my paraplegic condition resulting from a decades-long battle with multiple sclerosis.

Against the gripping fear of helplessness I struggled like a mackerel pulled out of the sea and tossed haphazardly on the surface of a slick fishing boat. Struggle is almost instinctive in times like these, though the biggest battles are internal. Like pride, even when it's wounded. *Especially* when it's wounded.

My wife and I tried for a long time to haul me up off the floor. Too long. Between my height and weight, the task was daunting—clearly a fool's errand. Yet, I insisted again and again that we could do it without anyone else's help. Maybe if she lifted under my arms and turned me onto my side? Maybe if I placed my neck on the pillow, she could drag me into the other room?

My body began to shake involuntarily—despite the blanket

I INSISTED
AGAIN AND AGAIN
THAT WE COULD
DO IT WITHOUT
ANYONE ELSE'S
HELP.

———————— ≋ ————————

she had placed over my drying frame—as that fear and frustration settled in like an early winter frost. Due to my condition, I already asked for so much help. Why couldn't I do something so simple—so terrifyingly simple—without calling for aid?

Finally, after needless tears and buckets of exasperation, we called my neighbor. Parley, a Vin Diesel doppelganger and no stranger to hardship himself, had offered us assistance many times, though I had always assured him we were fine. *Fine.* And we were. If lying on the floor naked, uninjured yet helpless—an embarrassing position for anyone to see me in—counted as *fine,* that is.

After our call for help, Parley arrived in moments with a wooden stool of his grandmother's and a diffusing and accepting joke, he found a way that neither my wife nor

I had thought of and put me back in my wheelchair in no time.

I realized then that I wasn't fine—hadn't been fine—and that, however much I didn't want to, it was time to ask for and receive help.

I have learned many hard lessons in recent years. One of them, for example, is that suffering is a skill. We can embrace pain. Buckets of pain. And, when we think we can't hold anymore, we can get a bigger bucket. But there will also be times when the pain flows over the edge, when the tub we have to hold life neatly together fails us, and it is in these moments we are invited to consider how vulnerable we are.

John Donne said it best in his famous ode to community and collected potential that "no man is an island"[1] which reminds us we are part of the main—part of the whole. I

IT IS IN THESE
MOMENTS
THAT WE ARE INVITED
TO CONSIDER HOW
VULNERABLE
WE ARE.

offer that each of us will be gifted to learn that there is an interconnectedness of humanity to catch us—if we will but ask.

Which brings me to perhaps the greatest lesson—the hardest lesson learned over the past years—*how to receive.*

When I say the word *receive*, what comes to mind? If you work in business, you may think of shipping and receiving. There are receiving lines at weddings, receiving blankets at baby showers, or wide receivers if you are a sports fan, key players on any football team. Whatever your initial thoughts were, let me ask the question:

What does it really mean to receive?

We don't spend too much time thinking about it. No one wants to be seen as weak, as a charity case, the drain on someone else's time or resources. Instead, we like the idea of being self-sufficient. Rugged individualists. Lone wolves. (Which is a misnomer, since wolves are actually pack animals.) We would far rather focus on giving than receiving.

As a Christ-centered people, we give service through countless acts on a regular basis and suffer our own pain in silence. We give plates of warm baked cookies, compliments, and platitudes. And this is commendable. Mostly. It's also an accepted rule of life: we lift others, thereby lifting ourselves. (Though, it turns out that *why* and *how* we do what we do is important. Motives matter.)

Think of the service you've given to others and how good you've felt afterwards. It has been shown that giving offers immediate paybacks with its own dopamine-induced euphoria known as the "helper's high."[2] According to some researchers, humans have an almost altruistic propensity toward these pro-social behaviors and their built-in chemical rewards.

Sometimes we do acts of service solely for self-serving reasons: it makes us feel good, plain and simple. I liken these times to being *nice.* These times don't have the same deeper payoffs we might think, though they look and feel good on the surface. We might, like Mr. Elton in a retelling of *Emma,* seek or appreciate the recognition we receive from our niceness. "Thank you," he says, after performing a menial task on Emma's behest, "for thinking me thoughtful."[3] As much as he loved his neighbors, he loved feeling good about serving them even more.

According to Buddhist teachings, "It's not how much you do for others, but the kindness you pour into it."[4] In one research study, we learn that life's longevity extends when our hearts are motivated by "kind giving" or "kind altruism."[5] So it appears there's a difference between being *nice* (surface) and *kind* (core). *Nice* is the equivalent, it turns out, as empty or no giving. Again, as simple as *giving* seems, motive matters.

Of course, not all support this thinking. Sartre and his ilk offer that anyone that's giving you something—regardless of their motive—is also trying to sell you something. Like the Brooklyn Bridge.[6] (Buyer beware!) Think *Lord of the Flies* by William Golding or Thomas Hobbes' proposition that we are naturally selfish.[7]

AGAIN
AS SIMPLE
AS GIVING
SEEMS, MOTIVE
MATTERS.

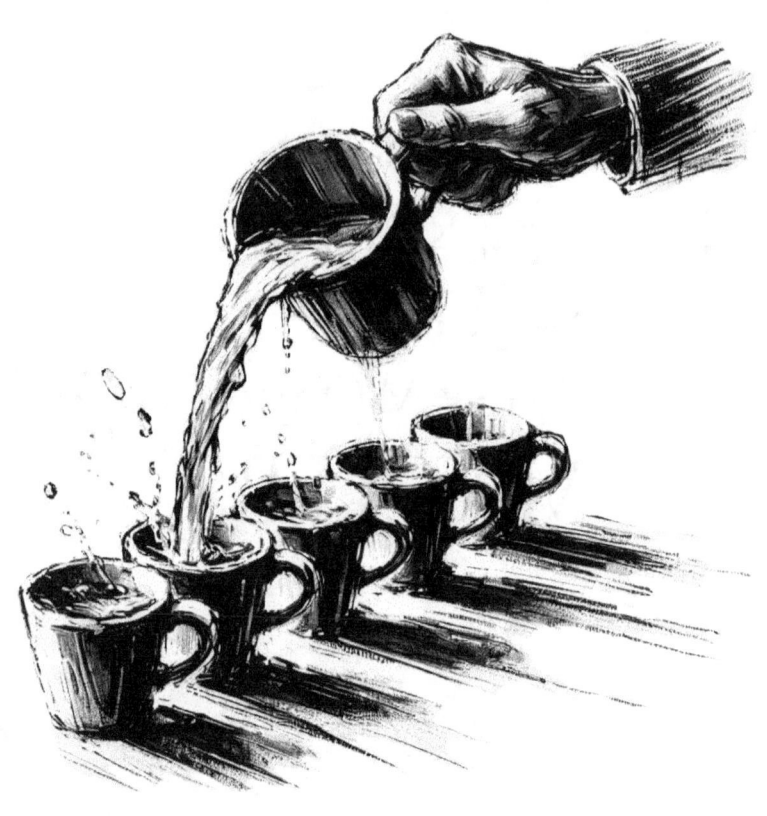

Nevertheless, still other studies show that kindness and giving benefits individuals *and* social groups, for we know that kindness has a cascading effect.[8] Regardless of which camp you hail from, there is little argument that giving [both the *nice* and *kind* iterations] is what we as a people do best. As mystifying as these simple acts can prove to be, I offer a shift in perspective here, *if you are willing to receive it.*

Perhaps as confusing as the concept of *receiving* itself, one of the greatly misunderstood scriptures is "...remember the words of the Lord Jesus, how he said, It is more blessed to give than to receive."[9] We may conclude from this verse that *giving* is better than *receiving*. Yet, as is true when cherry-picking from scripture, much is lost when this verse is read out of context.

These words are part of Paul's counsel to the elders of the church at Ephesus where he reminds these leaders to give *of their substance* to *the church* rather than receive *the substance of the church* unto themselves. But, as is true with hasty conclusions, it's easy to latch onto the last words and believe by overgeneralization that "it is more blessed to give than to receive." And, in our latching, we might endorse it as God's will. His edict. His command. Give, *give*, and give some more. Give until you feel like an empty well.

The problem here is that once we've given everything, there's nothing left to draw from, particularly if we've not yet learned to receive as the woman of Samaria received her Lord, the source of all living water.

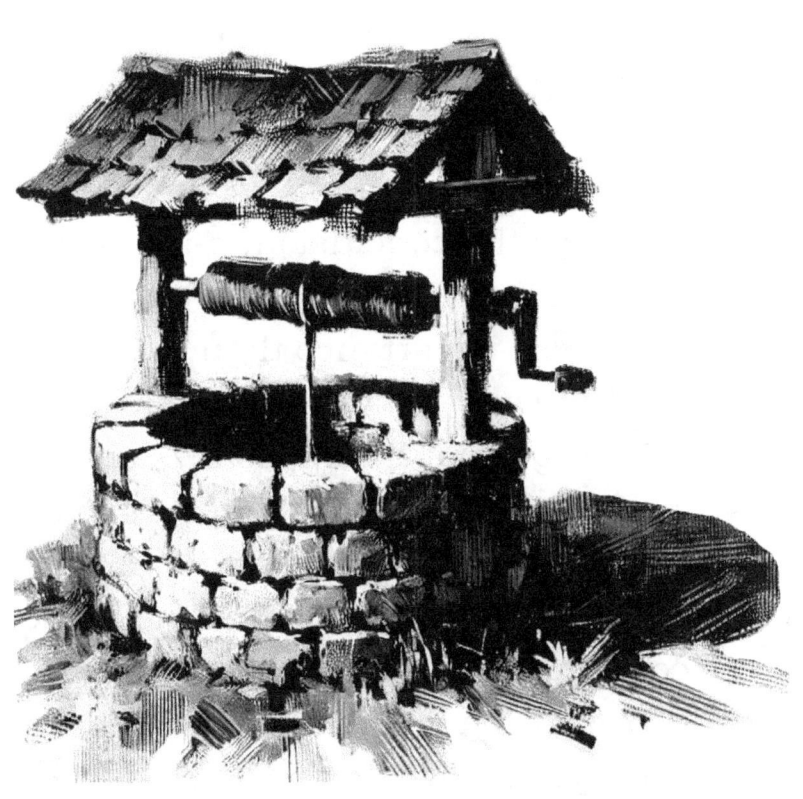

While the bible mentions the word *give* more than 2000 times, the word *receive* is mentioned on just over 300 occasions. From this disparate view, it's easy to think of the two concepts as being opposites. Surely the word mentioned most frequently must be the most important. We can easily arrive at the conclusion, once again, that receiving is a type of foil and is of far less importance than giving.

However, I would offer that *receiving* is not the opposite of giving. *Selfishness* is the opposite of giving. Giving and receiving are companions, two sides of the same coin, *inseparable*.

Yet even in our enlightened society, the well-suited duo is not regarded equally. We fear that asking for help—openly receiving from others—makes us moochers.

Freeloaders. Users. Ridiculous. Societal outcasts. Or worse, weak.

According to a study by the University of British Columbia, giving is considered pro-social behavior, whereas receiving is not.[10] The truth can be hard to discern with so many conflicting approaches, yet the wise author George MacDonald offers, "More important even than a knowledge of the truth is our willingness *to receive it.*"[11]

We can be given the world, we can be given the truth, we can be given hope, but *only if we receive it.* The willingness to *receive* is critical for every one of us. For example, Nephi reminds that "[The Lord gives] all things which man is prepared to receive."[12]

So, I ask again, what does it mean to *receive*? And how does one prepare to receive? I would offer that receiving means to accept, to allow ourselves to be blessed, *to be changed by the gift and by the giver.* Brene' Brown reminds us that "Until we can receive with an open heart, we're never really giving with an open heart. When we attach judgment to receiving help, we knowingly or unknowingly attach judgment to giving help."[13]

To prepare to receive something, we must first be open to change. Change in perspective. Change in attitude. Change from independence to interdependence.

Whenever something new is entertained as a possibility, something old passes away. That can be long held beliefs, or short-term judgments. As one author has said, "Receiving is death to the ego. It is total humility. It is the end of 'I am

MORE
IMPORTANT
EVEN THAN A
KNOWLEDGE OF THE
TRUTH IS OUR
WILLINGNESS
TO RECEIVE IT.

GENUINE
RECEIVING
REQUIRES A
WILLINGNESS TO BE
CHANGED FROM
OUR
EGOCENTRIC STATE
TO A STATE OF
HUMILITY.

———≈———

an independent person who can take care of myself.' To fully receive, a lot of stressful beliefs have to fall away."[14]

In sum, whenever we give, someone else receives. And that someone, whether they are conscious of it or not, agrees to be changed in some way because genuine giving calls for genuine receiving. (Note the *genuine* qualifier; disingenuity requires no such exchange as it remains a surface act.)

Genuine receiving requires a willingness to be changed from our egocentric state to a state of humility which is the antithesis of pride. Is it any wonder we struggle? To truly receive means we place a greater focus on the other person than on ourselves. Is this not a profound way to serve others?

Building on this idea, Elder Marion G. Romney adds that "Service [from others] is not something we endure on this earth so we can earn the right to live in the celestial kingdom. Service [received] is the very fiber of which an exalted life in the celestial kingdom is made."[15]

How can we possibly think that we are ready or able to receive something as grandiose as Eternal Life when we can scarcely receive compliments, gifts, or acts of service from our friends and neighbors? I implore you not to wait until you are naked and vulnerable to begin to understand and be blessed by the true gifts of receiving.

A modern parable, then, to consider.

There was a man who after many years of companionship lost his best

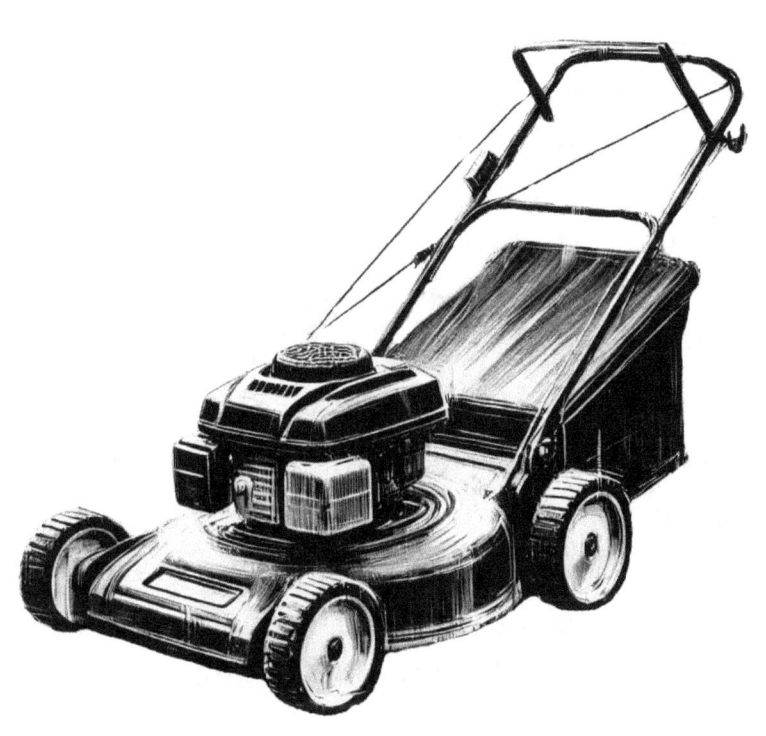

friend—his lawnmower. Upon reflection, the man decided to acquire a new machine, capable of improvements in both time and efficiency. Eager to not have the lawnmower sit idle for six days a week, the man inquired of his neighbors if he might be of service in mowing their lawns.

The first neighbor he approached thanked him for his desire but indicated that he was a self-proclaimed perfectionist and that his lawn needed to be mowed in a very specific way to be acceptable, something he did not even trust his married children to do. (Only his wife could do the job correctly.)

Undaunted, the lawnmower owner approached a second neighbor but was refused outright. "I am a capable man that can mow his own lawn—thank you, anyway."

Only slightly discouraged, he approached a third neighbor. The response surprised him again. "I know we are poor and only have a push mower to do the job, but we are not afraid of hard work, and on top of that my boy needs the exercise."

Enthusiasm waning in direct correlation to his rising discouragement, the man tried again and again to be of service. Responses were different but the result was the same: no lawn mowing.

"I pay someone to take care of it" said one.

"My lazy, good-for-nothing children will come any day to do their duty. Any day now," said another.

"I like the overgrowth; it reminds me of the country," said a third.

In the end, man and machine sat idle with all of the desire to serve but nowhere for that service to be rendered.

Is this parable difficult to believe, or do we think it would never happen in our own neighborhoods? I speak this parable from personal experience. When my boy was twelve years old, we thought to help him and his best friend understand the value of service. So, we loaded up their lawnmowers and tried to find someone who would receive them. Rejection after rejection left their lawnmowers unused. Only when they solicited money for their work were their services accepted.

Were the intended recipients bad people? Did they want to discourage and cause emotional harm to the boys? Very likely not. But they and our sons lost an important opportunity to serve and be served. They say the grass in your yard is only as green as you mow it. I wonder if it gets greener when we accept the service offered by others?

I would submit that—specifically in this situation—these neighbors *thought they were doing something noble* by refusing help. I am sure they felt self-reliant or capable themselves. For years I shared their same condition. I was fully capable, thank you very much. Until I wasn't. Until I couldn't even tie my own shoes. One of the unexpected gifts of my condition has been this shift in perspective.

As someone fully reliant as a receiver on the care and giving from others, I see things differently now.

We don't have to wait for a chronic illness to change our perspective, to recognize how much we're potentially missing out on. As shared in a conference talk, "One cannot help but wonder how many gifts and blessings surround us that we do not receive."[16]

In Romans we are told to "receive ye one another, as Christ also received us."[17] How is it that we focus on the giving aspect of the coin and ignore the receiving, though it, too, was modeled by the Lord? As we've been told, "Such receiving is a foundational gospel pattern. It is set forth in the very ordinance by which we are confirmed members of the Church. In this ordinance, we are instructed to 'receive the Holy Ghost.' This is a formal invitation to act, to receive this great gift."[18]

Other examples include our willingness to receive the name of Christ by partaking of the sacrament: "that they are willing to take upon them," the scripture states.[19] Are we willing?

Furthermore, Elder David A. Bednar offers that "The Holy Ghost does not become operative in our lives merely because hands are placed upon our heads and those four important words are spoken. ... These four words—'Receive the Holy Ghost'—are not a passive pronouncement; rather, they constitute a priesthood injunction—an authoritative admonition to act and not simply to be acted upon.

As we receive this ordinance, each of us accepts a sacred and ongoing responsibility to desire, to seek, to work, and to so live that we indeed "receive the Holy Ghost" and its attendant spiritual gifts. "For what doth it profit a man if a gift is bestowed upon him, and he receive not the gift? Behold, he rejoices not in that which is given unto him, neither rejoices in him who is the giver of the gift."[20]

He also offers that "A teacher can explain, demonstrate, persuade, and testify, and do so with great spiritual power and effectiveness. Ultimately, however, the content of a message and the witness of the Holy Ghost penetrate into the heart only if a receiver allows them to enter."[21]

As suggested, the scriptures are replete with pleas, invitations, and examples of receiving. I offer only a few here:

"How oft I would have gathered you as a hen gathereth her chicks...and ye would not."[22]

"He that is built upon the rock receiveth it."[23]

"He that is able to receive it, let him receive it."[24]

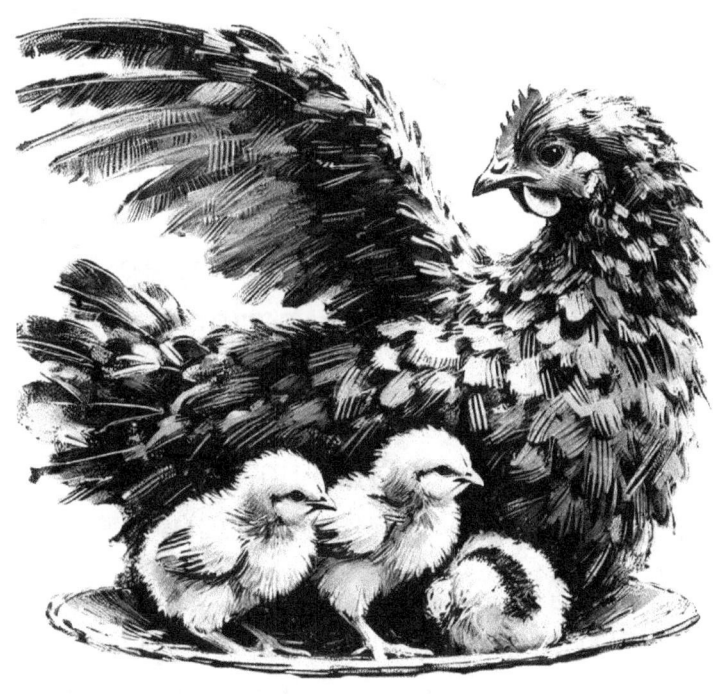

"He that receiveth light and continueth in light receiveth more light."[25]

"None receiveth save it be the truly penitent and humble seeker of happiness."[26]

And, we've heard the scripture that everyone appreciates a cheerful giver.[27] What of the receiver? Are they not equally appreciated? Perhaps a deeper dive into the scriptures is warranted. As stated by Elder Roger Merrill: "As I have become more aware of this principle, I find that the scriptures are replete with the doctrine of receiving."[28]

How willing we are to receive affects every aspect of our lives—our work, our spouses, our children, our friends, ourselves. Every saving ordinance of the church involves receiving on our part. When we receive the sacrament, we are not taking from the Savior; we are accepting the gift and the associated covenants and allowing our lives to be changed. Answers to prayer come when we're ready to receive them.

Though the word receive appears only 300 times in scripture, the concept of an open mind and heart, of a willing disposition, of a prepared soil awaiting the Sower, permeates doctrinal teachings. As President Boyd K. Packer has said, "No message appears in scripture more times, in more ways than, 'Ask, and ye shall receive.'"[29] Clearly, *receiving* is a foundational gospel pattern. At the very core of our mortal probation is the choice to receive.

How many blessings pass us by because we are unwilling to ask for what we need?

In church meetings, in personal and family scripture study, and even this day as you're reading these words, some will receive more than others. Why? I am learning that those who truly receive do at least three things that others may not.

First, they seek. We live in a consumer world, a spectator world. We seek to be entertained. "Is it fun?" we ask at every turn. "Is it easy?" Without realizing it, we can find ourselves coming to church with the attitude, "Here I am; now, inspire me." We become spiritually passive. When we focus instead on seeking and receiving the pearls through the Holy Ghost, we become less concerned about a teacher or speaker holding our attention and more concerned about giving our attention to the Spirit.

Remember, *receive* is a verb. The other side of the giving coin. It is a

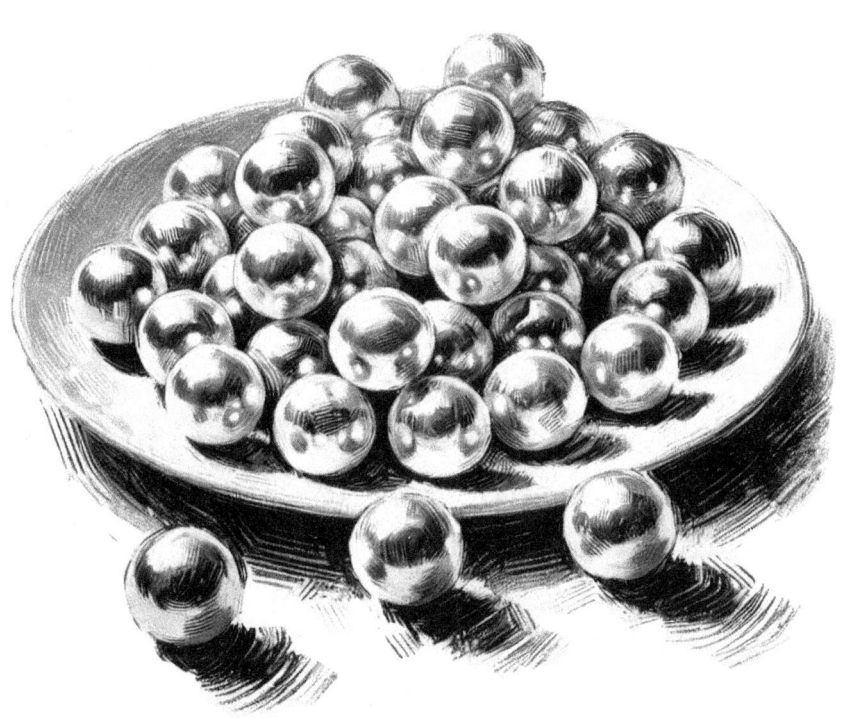

principle of action. It is a fundamental expression of faith.

Second, those who receive, *feel.* While revelation comes to the mind and heart, it is also often felt. Until we learn to pay attention to these spiritual feelings, we often fail to recognize the promptings of the Spirit. We can be like Amulek who said, *"I knew concerning these things, yet I would not know..."*[30]

Third, those who receive by the Spirit intend to act. As the prophet Moroni instructed, to receive a witness of the Book of Mormon, we must ask "with real intent."[31] It can be easy to think this verse is referring to an intent to *know. Please, Lord,* we pray, *I really, really, want to know...*

While that may be partially true, I've wondered if this injunction isn't

RECEIVING IS A FOUNDATIONAL GOSPEL PATTERN.

———— ≋ ————

also inviting us *to act*: to pray with real intent to act on the answers we may receive, and to change our lives in whatever way may be needed—in whatever "knowing" may require.

What if the Spirit teaches when we honestly intend to do something about what we learn? Being a good receiver is the key to continued light and knowledge.

The Prophet Joseph Smith gently reprimanded, "I could explain a hundredfold more than I ever have... were I permitted, and were the people ready to receive them. The Lord deals with this people as a tender parent with a child, communicating light and intelligence and the knowledge of His ways as they can bear it."[32]

Note the Prophet's response in the following oft-quoted experience that Brother Brigham had in a dream with Brother Joseph. Keep in mind that Brother Brigham was considered "the Lion of the Lord."

"'Brother Joseph, the brethren ... have a great anxiety to understand the ... sealing principles; and if you have a word of counsel for me, I should be glad to receive it.' As a piece of what Joseph replied, "Tell the brethren to keep their hearts open to conviction, so that when the Holy Ghost comes to them, their hearts will be ready to receive it."[33]

Here we learn another piece to the puzzle: to "keep [our] hearts open to conviction" as preparation for receiving greater light and knowledge. Keeping an open heart when we are bombarded daily by tremendous onslaughts through social media and news teeming with fabrications and half-truths, as well

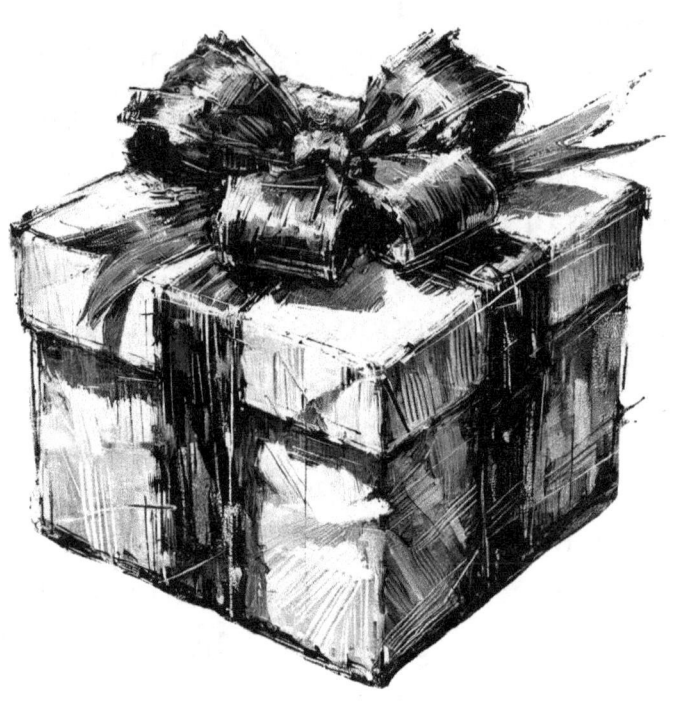

as our own internal fears and anxieties, can prove a daunting task. As Luke reminds, "Men's hearts [will fail] them for fear, and for looking after those things which are coming on the earth: for the powers of heaven shall be shaken."[34]

Being open to receiving represents the ultimate vulnerability with the potential for pain, disappointment, and unmet expectations. Rejection also looms as a real possibility when what is given is not what we expect or maybe even want. As mentioned earlier, in our modern day we may even think that receiving is synonymous with taking, and that the giver is left with less.

When my wife Paulette was on her mission in England, she met a young Turkish woman attending a singles' ward there. With a marked kindness to others, Nareen was lovely inside and out. When Paulette finally worked up the courage and complimented her by stating that she was a beautiful person, Nareen reached out and taking Paulette's hand in hers, responded by saying, "Oh, sister, it is because of the beauty in you that you see it so readily in others." Paulette was stunned speechless by Nareen's response. Such grace. Such *receiving*.

Nareen did not refute the compliment but accepted it with humility. Forty years later Nareen's words still resonate as an example my wife seeks to emulate.

I suspect that most of us when we receive a compliment are more likely to discount it and thereby discount the giver, as well. After speaking in church, for example, you might say,

"Brother Kirkham, you gave a good talk today." And, in the past, I have said things like "It was nothing." (Also meaning the compliment was nothing or that the giver of the compliment was nothing.) Or I may have drawn even more attention to myself by saying, "I'm not a very good speaker" or "I get nervous talking in church." These responses, though common and understandable, inadvertently discount both the compliment and the giver. (Please note how many times I said "I" in those previous examples.)

My personal experience in this area is that giving is rarely a problem; it is in the receiving where we fall short.

In the scenario above, imagine grace coming into the exchange instead of insecurity or egoism. When we're complimented, we receive it with "Thanks for sharing that" or "That means a lot coming from you." Grace would join both the giver and the receiver for a moment in time.

Grace is in low supply in our modern exchanges, isn't it? When we are unwilling to receive, we unwittingly put up a wall that prevents the potential for real connection. How can others feel close to us when we keep the castle turrets, towers, and battlements so strongly guarded?

A simple first step might be, when complimented, to try avoiding downplaying, deflecting, or putting yourself down. As shared by an executive training company, "Can you imagine refusing to receive a gift from someone you care about? Well, that's essentially what you are doing when you reject a compliment. Not only does it make you seem ungrateful, but it is also insulting and dismissive to the person offering the praise. My mother taught me that the most gracious way to accept a gift I didn't expect (or want) is just to say "thank you" and zip it!"[35]

Grace can be challenging whether we're receiving a compliment or giving a gift of our own. Many times in my own experience and in the experience of others I've spoken with, receivers do not always receive well, either ignoring the offering, escalating the gift giving, or outright rejecting the compliment or gift.

Some of us have the mistaken belief that it's selfish to receive, that we don't deserve someone else's affection or attention, or that we must one-up or reciprocate. Sometimes we think in a "tit for tat" mindset, realizing that we can't

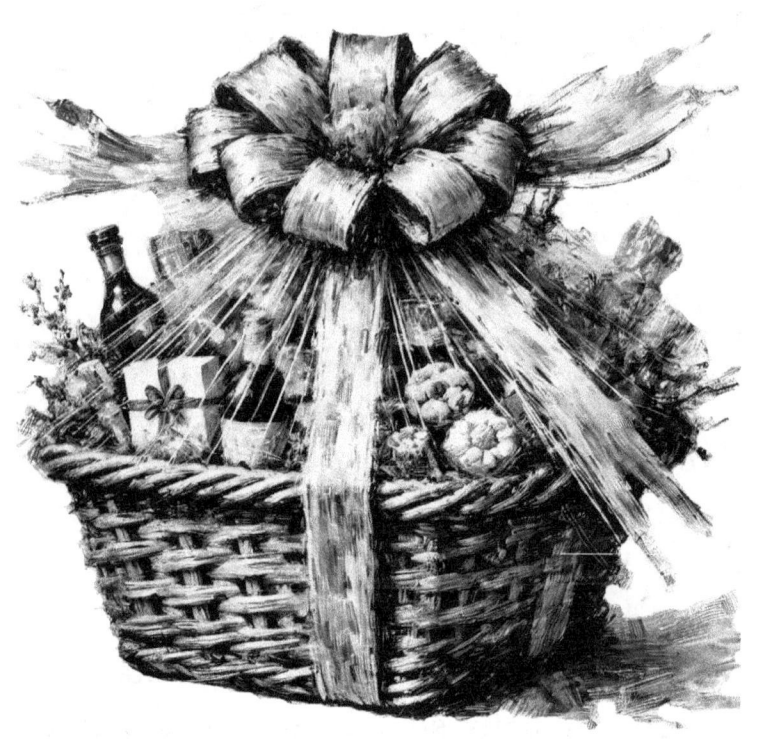

afford to give back in equal measure, or we resist because we feel there are strings attached to the giving. And sometimes there are. Regardless of our thoughts---some justified from negative experiences, perhaps---the end result is pushing others and their gifts away diminishing the giving and receiving.

There was a time in my life when I was proud of the fact that I could not be "out given." If someone gave me a gift, I would give a better one back. I was not to be outdone, and I would be in no one's debt. What do you think happened? My opportunities to give dried up. No one was willing to give to me because of the consequences of doing so, and who would receive from me when an escalation was expected? I had no grace and no understanding of what receiving and true giving was.

Are we one-uppers? Do we "get people back" when they give to us, escalating a cycle of giving with the need to be the "best givers"? Let us not mistake our gratitude for service as a reason to "out-do" those who have given to us. I have learned through long experience that there is no way to repay—our gratitude is all we really have to give. Giving with no strings attached is equally as important as receiving with no strings attached.

I have need to heed my own counsel more than most of you, I suspect. As you can see by my condition, confined as I am to a wheelchair, I believe that my ability to give is diminishing as my need to receive increases. I have felt in the past that somehow the two balance each other out or that I must give more than I receive somehow to be of societal worth.

While I can understand the falseness of this assumption intellectually, accepting the reality of it is a very different matter.

One of my greatest fears has been to need help from someone else, to require service from another's hand to eat, to shower, to live, to be unable to do the things that "real men" do. That fear has at times overtaken me. I struggle regularly with my inadequacy as a husband, father, and friend due to my perceived inability to throw down my "man card" and be the giver all the time.

Be that as it may, without the events in my life and where they have led me, I would have had no real reason to change. No reason to obtain characteristics of godliness. How would I have had the desire to

HOW WOULD I HAVE
HAD THE DESIRE TO
BECOME MEEK AND
LOWLY OF HEART
WERE IT NOT FOR MY
PRESENT STATE?

become meek and lowly of heart were it not for my present state?

Perhaps it would be helpful when talking about receiving to clarify the difference between *giving* and *getting*.

When we give with expectations about exactly what it is we want to give with no regard for what the recipient requires, the gift becomes more about getting than giving. From the beginning the gift is about our desires, not those of the intended recipient. The husband, who gives his wife a griddle for her birthday because he wants pancakes, has given himself a gift, not his wife. Had she given him the griddle for his birthday, with its implied promise, it would have been a true gift. As it was, the husband might have given himself a checkmark for a gift that was only "a get."

With gifts, there may also come expectations as we receive them. Where is the line between being a grateful receiver and an entitled taker? The key is in assuming that a gift given is deserved in the first place—that we are entitled to our needs being prioritized and met. Are we?

At what point does the gift of being moved from the bed to my wheelchair no longer warrant gratitude? Every instance of a need met invites reciprocating grace, for are we not all beggars?[36]

Again, how can any giving occur if there is no one willing to receive?

A former relief society president in a neighboring stake in Rexburg said that on any given day, if she had a sign-up sheet and asked for volunteers to help others—in other words, to *give*—it would be filled within a matter of minutes; but, were she to ask for sign-ups from people who would be willing to receive—the sheet would come back empty. What are we afraid of? Are we afraid of appearing less than self-sufficient, competent, or in control?

How many of us keep our friends, neighbors, and home ministers at arm's length when they ask what they can do and we say, "If something comes up, I'll let you know"?

Do we show our unwillingness to receive what is offered from a relief society activity involving a craft by not attending at all?

Having served as an elders quorum president on a few occasions, I understand that elders quorums may have a reputation for

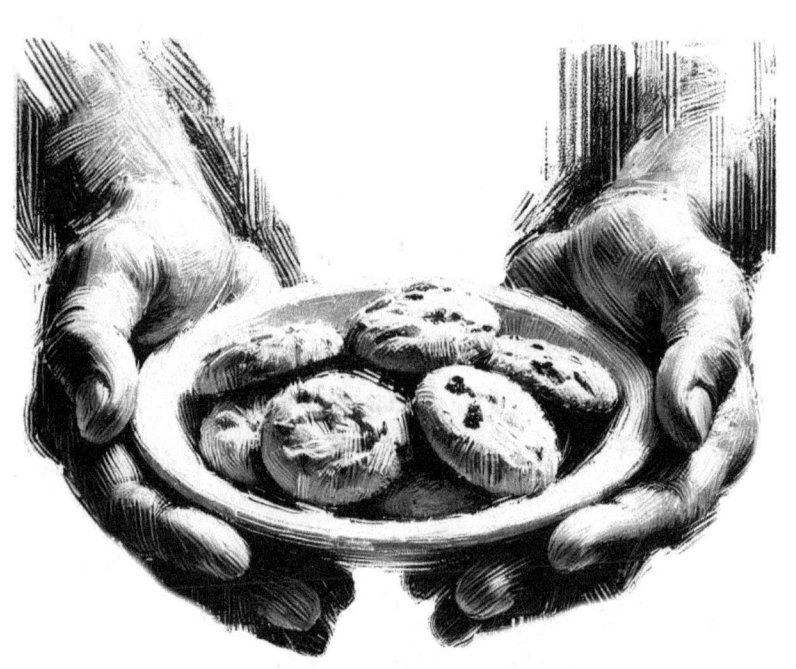

performing work that might not meet code or require some touch up afterwards. I could share some stories with you that might confirm your worst fears, but I'll save those for another time; however, will we rob them of their giving because we are not capable of receiving what is being offered?

Can you imagine the surprise on the faces of your home ministers if you actually asked for help with some simple tasks when they offered their services? It only takes moments to wipe some counters, grab the mail, put a few dishes away, or sweep a porch. These simple acts of service can build lasting bridges while teaching us how to receive through modest baby steps.

Several years ago, my roof found itself in need of replacement. The roofer we had chosen offered to reduce the price if I would remove the old roof rather than having them do it. The option was attractive, but my first thoughts were, 'The last thing I want to do is burden someone with the task of working on my roof on a Friday night.' That thought gave way to, 'Who would even show up? Surely people have other things to do.' And then I thought, 'It is worth the extra money to have someone else deal with it than to make the effort to coordinate an event.'

My wife was undeterred and took the roofer's offer.

Later, when we were alone, I expressed my misgivings. "Unless you have a thirty-foot-long scraper with a wheelchair attachment, you and the kids are going to be on the roof for a week trying to get that job done." Her response was faithful in

THESE SIMPLE ACTS
OF SERVICE CAN BUILD
LASTING BRIDGES
WHILE TEACHING
US HOW TO RECEIVE
THROUGH MODEST
BABY STEPS.

———— ≈ ————

contrast to my incredulity. "They will come," she said.

The appointed time came, and I struggled with an "I told you so" when only two people arrived, but I held my tongue—and was glad that I did, for within the fifteen minutes of what we call Mormon Standard Time two wards worth of elders, high priests, and their families arrived and finished that massive job in less than two hours. As the event was coming to a close, one of the bishops who was present said to me in passing, "We need more things like this around here. So many are willing, able, and even excited to have an opportunity to serve yet so few are willing to accept that service."

This is but one example of the enormous giving on my behalf from my ward and stake. I could scarcely name them all: the people and the service: shoveling, painting, sanding, raking, fixing, baking, cleaning, and so much more. Countless and boundless giving. And, as a grateful receiver, I have been moved. Humbled. *Changed.*

Now, I will be the first to say that receiving can be hard. I think it is even harder when the situation has the potential to be embarrassing, like the floor incident I opened these thoughts with. My pride was of no service or value to me that day. Only my willingness to receive was what saved me (and a really strong friend, I must say.) Clearly, it would have been foolish for me to continue to say, "No, no, I got this. I can do this myself. I don't need any help."

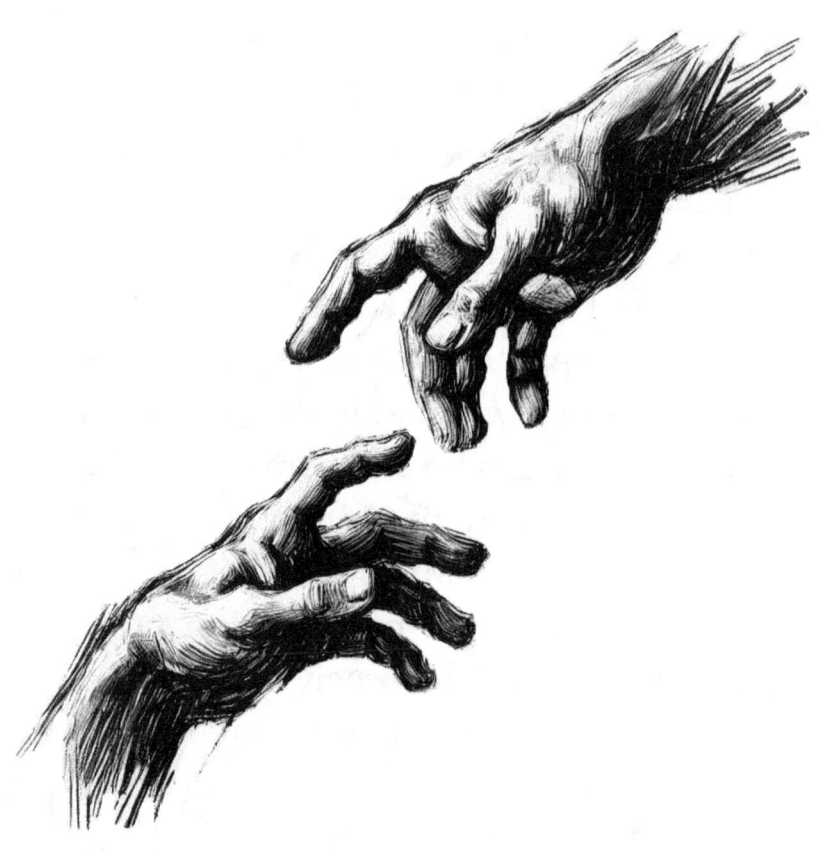

You may see yourself like you are the exception and really don't—or won't—ever need help. We all need help, if not today then perhaps tomorrow. When your time of need arises, and it will, rest assured that our Father in Heaven has already gone ahead to spread the table of provision on your behalf, if you are willing to receive it.[37] Christ stands at the door, ready for us to knock.

Let's give up our foolish pride and express our needs to those who have stewardship over us. Give your family, friends, roommates, and home ministers an opportunity to bring the considerable power of the fellowship of the saints to bear on your behalf. Even if the task seems small or embarrassing, I invite all to give someone the opportunity to give by expressing a need to receive.

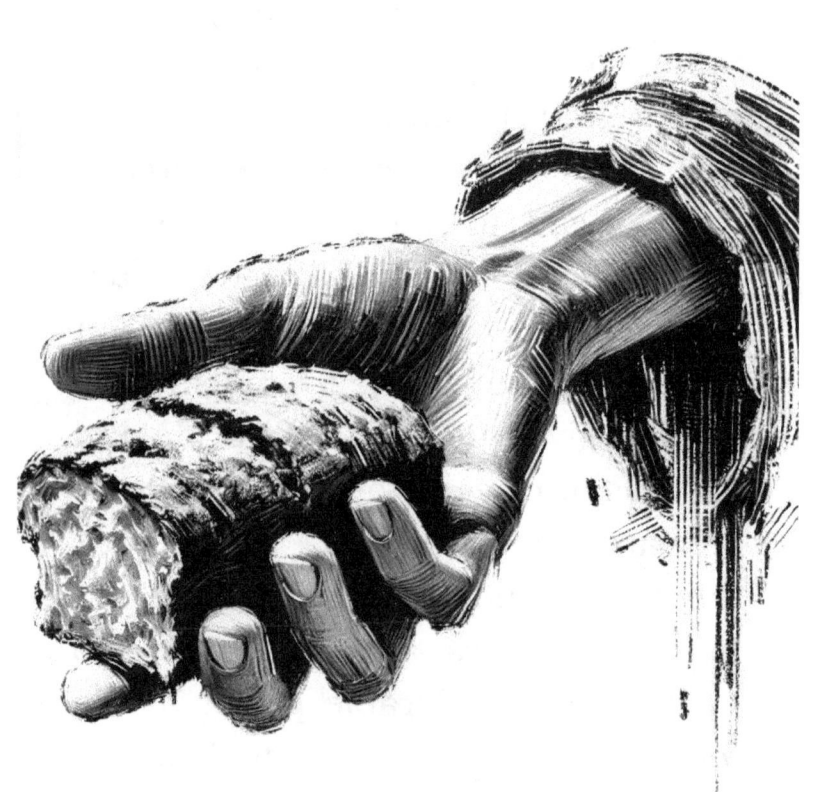

When the call comes, be a part of the giving when it is needed, for giving is one of the things that we do best as a people, as a community, and as disciples of Christ.

Then, when we are ready, we can open our hearts to the gifts that our Father in Heaven and our Savior have waiting for us—if we are only willing to receive them.

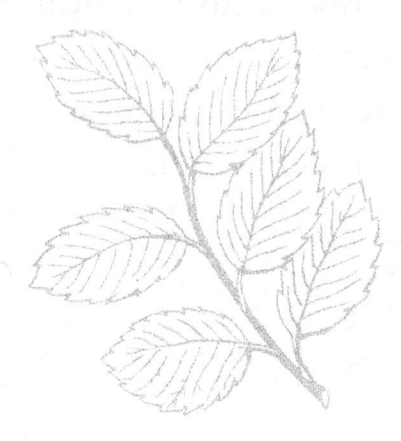

I'm a novice when it comes to receiving.
Giving has become my second expertise,
But giving alone without getting
Soon becomes a fatal disease.

If the intake valve is not opened
There's no way to maintain a supply
There comes a point in the cycle of life
Where the out-going stream runs dry.

Straining out love from a vacuum
Is like drinking from the heart of a stone.
Try as we may, at the end of the day,
We're exhausted, frustrated, and alone.

'Better to give than to receive', we are taught
Yet another truth I've learnt just by living:
Only the soul with the grace to receive,
Excels in the fine art of giving.

- Dr. James A. Forbes Jr.[38]

ABOUT THE AUTHOR

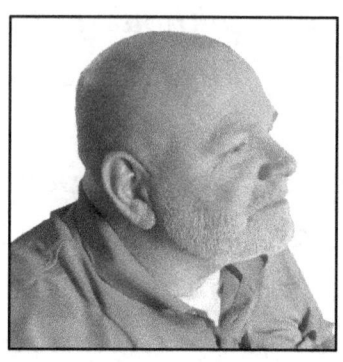

Drake Kirkham spent many years dodging opportunities to receive— until his MS diagnosis invited him to consider another alternative. He's grateful to pay some small part of his experience forward.

When he isn't pondering the mysteries of faith and personal commitment to a loving Savior, he enjoys reading literature and popcorn fiction, learning through courses taken through the Jordan

Peterson Academy, and emerging triumphant in bitter battles for LOTR Settlers of Catan, Scrabble, and Klank titles.

A rich surprise has come through the concourse of lives that have intersected with his through various Tuesday's With Morrie moments. Drake also enjoys maintaining good relationships with his favorite son, Quinn, his favorite daughter, Aubrey, and a multiplicity of enthusiastic grandchildren.

Last, but certainly not least, Drake treasures his lifetime companion and beautiful gift, Paulette, who aided him in the editing and production of this manuscript.

He also helped in his career to send things to Mars. No big deal.

ENDNOTES

[1] "No Man is An Island" by John Donne from "Devotions upon Emergent Occasions" (1624). "No man is an island, Entire of itself, Every man is a piece of the continent, A part of the main. If a clod be washed away by the sea, Europe is the less. As well as if a promontory were. As well as if a manor of thy friend's Or of thine own were: Any man's death diminishes me, Because I am involved in mankind, And therefore never send to know for whom the bell tolls; It tolls for thee."

[2] The Healing Power of Doing Good by Allan Luks. Luks's purpose is to show exactly how one's physical health, not just emotional well-being, is improved through helping others.

[3] Emma by Jane Austen, 1815. Austen is widely known for her witty—and accurate—social insights and critiques.

[4] "What We Get When We Give" by Molly McDonough. Harvard Medicine. https://magazine.hms.harvard.edu/articles/what-we-get-when-we-give. "A few years ago, a small study from an international research collaboration that included scientists from the National Institutes of Health used magnetic resonance imaging to measure brain activity associated with making a charitable donation. The findings, reported in PNAS, suggested that this action engages the mesolimbic system of the brain, triggering a euphoric rush of dopamine in much the same way that anticipating a reward, like money, does."

[5] Blueprint: The Evolutionary Origins of a Good Society by Nicholas Christakis. "A dazzlingly erudite synthesis of history, philosophy, anthropology, genetics, sociology, economics, epidemiology, statistics, and more" (Frank Bruni, The New York Times).

[6] In the early 1900s, George Parker mastered the art of selling New York landmarks that he didn't own, thus the colloquial reference of "If you believe that,

I've got a Brooklyn Bridge for sale, too."

[7] Leviathan by Thomas Hobbes (1651). In his famous work, Hobbes argues that people are inherently wicked and selfish, and he puts forth his ideas for the social contract and laws required by a society of evil creatures.

[8] Blueprint: The Evolutionary Origins of a Good Society by Nicholas Christakis

[9] The Bible, KJV, Acts 20:35

[10] "Prosocial Spending and Happiness: Using Money to Benefit Others Pays Off" by Dunn et al. "Although a great deal of research has shown that people with more money are somewhat happier than are people with less money, our research demonstrates that how people spend their money also matters for their happiness. In particular, both correlational and experimental studies have shown that people who spend money on others report more happiness. The benefits of such prosocial spending emerge among adults around the world, and the warm glow of giving can be detected even in toddlers. These benefits are most likely to emerge when giving satisfies one or more core human needs (relatedness, competence, and autonomy). The rewards of prosocial spending are observable in both the brain and the body and can potentially be harnessed by organizations and governments."

[11] The Truth by George Macdonald (1867). George MacDonald was the pioneer of modern fantasy. Influenced by his Scottish storytelling culture and Christian background, he created books that encouraged imagination. While his name might not be as well known, he went on to inspire two of the most famous fantasy writers of all time—J. R. R. Tolkien and C.S. Lewis.

[12] The Book of Mormon, 1 Nephi 17:30

[13] The Gifts of Imperfection by Brené Brown

[14] The Work as Meditation by Todd Smith. https://www.theworkasmeditation.com/2018/12/23/the-gift-of-receiving/

[15] Elder Marion G. Romney, Conference Report

"Gratitude and Thanksgiving," October 1982

[16] Elder A. Roger Merrill, Conference Report, "Receiving by the Spirit," October 2006

[17] The Bible, KJV, Romans 15:7

[18] Elder A. Roger Merrill, Conference Report, "Receiving by the Spirit," October 2006. "I have come to better understand how vitally important it is to receive by the Spirit. We often focus, appropriately, on the importance of teaching by the Spirit. But we need to remember that the Lord has placed equal, if not greater, importance on receiving by the Spirit." (See D&C 50:17–22.)

[19] Ibid

[20] Elder David A. Bednar, "Receive the Holy Ghost," October 2010

[21] Elder David A. Bednar, "Seek Learning by Faith," September 2007

[22] The Bible, KJV, Matthew 23:37

[23] The Bible, KJV, Matthew 7:24, 25

[24] The Bible, KJV, Matthew 19:12

[25] Doctrine and Covenants 50:24

[26] The Book of Mormon, Alma 27:18

[27] The Bible, KJV, 2 Corinthians 9:7

[28] Elder A. Roger Merrill, Conference Report, "Receiving by the Spirit," October 2006

[29] Elder Boyd K. Packer, Conference Report, "Reverence Invites Revelation," October 1991

[30] The Book of Mormon, Alma 10:5,6

[31] The Book of Mormon, Moroni 10:4

[32] Joseph Smith, Manuscript History of the Church, vol. D-1, page 1556, josephsmithpapers.org

[33] Brigham Young, https://sunstone.org/wp-content/uploads/sbi/articles/097-86.pdf

[34] The Bible, KJV, Luke 21:26

[35] "Can't Take a Compliment? How to Accept Praise More Gracefully," Jill Lynch Cruz. https://www.jlc.consulting/post/accept-praise-more-gracefully

[36] The Book of Mormon, Mosiah 4:16-19

[37] The Book of Mormon, 2 Nephi 32:5,6; Alma 13:1, Alma 32:27, Alma 37:13, Ether 12:9, Moroni 7:33

[38] Re. Dr. James A. Forbes Jr. 1995, New York City on Hendrix and Lakelly Hunt, 2004. Forbes was the recipient of fourteen honorary degrees, including D.D. degrees from Princeton University, Trinity

College, Colgate University, and University of Richmond. In 1996, Newsweek recognized Forbes as one of the twelve "most effective preachers" in the English-speaking world.

www.ingramcontent.com/pod-product-compliance
Lightning Source LLC
Chambersburg PA
CBHW070808120626
46557CB00002B/761